A MED

# A MEDICAL CATECHISM

**John Rees**
MD, MRCP

Consultant Physician and Senior Lecturer in Medicine,
Guy's Hospital Medical School, London

## HODDER AND STOUGHTON
LONDON SYDNEY AUCKLAND TORONTO

British Library CIP Data

Rees, John, *1949-*
  A medical catechism.
  1. Diagnosis
  I. Title
  616.07'5    RC71

ISBN 0 340 37676 7

First published 1986
Copyright © 1986 P. John Rees

Typeset by Rowland Phototypesetting Ltd,
Bury St Edmunds, Suffolk

Printed in Great Britain for Hodder and Stoughton Educational,
a division of Hodder and Stoughton Ltd,
Mill Road, Dunton Green, Sevenoaks, Kent TN13 2YD,
by Richard Clay Ltd, Bungay, Suffolk

# CONTENTS

# INTRODUCTION

Clinical skills involve the interpretation of accurate information in the history and examination with reference to the situation of a particular patient. This short book leads the medical student through all the aspects of the medical consultation and includes advice on case presentation. It stresses the importance of good communication in developing a rapport with the patient. In examination it aims to produce a reliable technique the results of which can be interpreted with confidence.

The book is aimed primarily at the new clinical student but provides valuable advice for all those faced with clerking patients and presenting their findings in ward rounds and examinations.

# THE RIGHT APPROACH

Much of the information doctors obtain from patients is of a very personal nature and patients will impart this freely only if they have confidence in their doctor. This involves having trust not only in the doctor's medical ability but also in his integrity, sympathy, interest and total discretion. Medical students need to develop the skills to put over these qualities to the patient and some find this difficult. It can be learnt by watching good doctors at work and also through practice. Not all doctors are good communicators and a critical selective approach to such learning is necessary, just as in lectures and when reading books and journals.

Students often feel vulnerable because they lack knowledge and experience and this may make them insecure in their early contact with patients. Avoid the easy response of being flippant or superficial and learn to develop a professional, caring attitude to your patients. This professional attitude extends to broader aspects of medicine. Rapid advances are being made in all fields of medicine and doctors owe it to their patients to develop a critical, enquiring mind to keep abreast of changes in the ethics and the science of medicine. This attitude is best established during student years.

Recording your findings following a clinical examination is an important part of patient care. Notes must always be comprehensive and legible to allow other health workers to retrieve relevant information. Communication with other doctors should be prompt and precise. The major message from the medical defence societies is that many of the legal problems increasingly associated with today's medicine could be avoided by adequate medical records.

Information about patients is confidential. This confidentiality is part of the contract between a patient and his doctor or medical student and the information should not be transmitted elsewhere without the informed consent of the patient.

# COMMUNICATION

The most common complaints about doctors and hospitals relate to failures in communication. Doctors and students are busy people but there must always be time to talk to the client. Giving the impression that you have time to talk is part of the effective 'bedside manner' thought by many patients and doctors to be neglected in today's training. Bear in mind that patients often remember little of what is told them at one consultation. They will remember more if given time to ask questions in a relaxed manner, less if a grand white-coated figure pontificates from the end of the bed while they lie exposed in ill-fitting hospital pyjamas with no buttons. Talk to patients on their level, physically and intellectually, in an unhurried way and with as much privacy as possible. Always be prepared to come back to reinforce any messages and answer any new questions and remember that you will encounter patients from many different social and cultural backgrounds.

During history taking, non-verbal communication is also important. This information will be missed if the history is taken while writing furiously in the notes and not observing the patient. Look at facial expressions, posture and evidence of agitation during the account. Let patients tell their own stories with occasional encouragement to show that it is what you want to hear. Develop your techniques for this encouragement and for leading patients away from irrelevant information back on to the right track. This is done by practice, by watching experienced interviewers and by watching your own technique on videotape.

Some situations provide particular communication difficulties, especially dealing with patients and relatives in cases of terminal disease. Videotapes and role-playing can help the student to work out his own attitude to such situations. An unhurried approach is even more important here, giving the patient time to ask questions and to return for further discussions.

Do not be afraid of physical contact; holding the patient's hand or arm may help him and show your sympathy and support.

# THE HISTORY

The history is the most important part of a consultation. Most diagnoses are made from the history and only confirmed or quantified on examination. Keep the history and examination separate. If the patient insists on showing some physical sign during the history do not dismiss it but show interest and reassure the patient that you will examine it fully after you have obtained the complete story.

Try to let the patient tell the story in his own words. Some will need prompting and directing more than others. Avoid leading questions to ensure that the patient decides for himself what he wants to say and does not just say what he thinks you want to hear.

Start the interview with some prior knowledge of the patient, at least name and age. Introduce yourself and take up a position close to the patient, not separated by a bed or desk. This helps to develop rapport between doctor and patient and will bring benefits in the history, examination and in subsequent treatment.

The history seeks information about symptoms. These are conditions of, or changes in, the body or its function which the patient perceives as abnormal or distressing. This is an important point. We generally deal with the patient's perception of reality as much as our own 'objective' reality, which relies on medical experience and an outsider's appreciation of the patient's feelings.

This history is divided into:

1 History of present complaint
2 Previous medical history
3 Routine review
4 Family history
5 Social history

The order of sections may vary but always starts with the current problem. Do not expect to get the story in perfect order. The patient may give relevant information at any time in the history. Keep good contact with the patient by restricting note-taking to a few salient points and dates, then write a full history afterwards.

Although the questions should be kept open, most doctors work by constructing possible hypotheses and testing these out during the history. Do not narrow your options too early but keep thinking and developing ideas while the patient is giving his history.

## HISTORY OF PRESENT COMPLAINT

Begin with the symptoms which caused the patient to seek medical help. Take the story through from the start of these complaints to the present. Then it will usually be necessary to obtain further information about the onset of the illness (e.g. 'when were you last quite well?') or about details of symptoms mentioned in the story.

Do not accept diagnoses from the patient without good evidence. Find out the symptoms instead. Make sure the patient understands the terms you are using, e.g. palpitations are interpreted in different ways by different patients.

Certain symptoms need to be qualified in standard ways. For example, with pain, find out:

**site**
**duration**
**character**
**severity**
**radiation**
**precipitating and relieving factors**
**pattern**

Quantify symptoms such as shortness of breath by reference to everyday tasks, such as walking upstairs or dressing.

In complicated histories go back over the story in such terms as 'As I understand what you have told me . . .'. This brings out any misunderstandings and often reminds the patient of other important facts.

## PREVIOUS MEDICAL HISTORY

The form of the previous medical history varies with the patient and the circumstances. In a ten year old boy with a fever, ask about previous infectious diseases and immunisations, but these questions will not be relevant to a 70 year old woman with chest pain.

In chest illnesses ask about previous X-rays, in heart disease ask about rheumatic fever and previous pregnancies, if applicable. With conditions such as rheumatic fever make sure the patient understands what you are asking.

Find out about previous operations, hospital admissions and other serious illnesses. List them with their dates and durations. Be careful about accepting the patient's diagnostic label for previous illnesses.

## ROUTINE REVIEW OF SYSTEMS

This section checks for other symptoms not covered in the main complaint. Explain that this is a routine list of questions. Most doctors develop their own list with experience.

A comprehensive starting list is:

1 GENERAL HEALTH

2 GASTROINTESTINAL

appetite
weight
nausea
vomiting
dysphagia
heartburn
abdominal pain
bowel habit—frequency
        —recent
            change
rectal bleeding, melaena

3 CARDIOVASCULAR

chest pain
palpitations
exercise tolerance
    (angina, dyspnoea)
orthopnoea
claudication
ankle swelling

4 RESPIRATORY

cough
sputum (colour, volume)
haemoptysis
wheeze

5 URINARY

frequency (nocturia)
stream (hesitancy,
    dribbling)
dysuria
haematuria
incontinence

6 SKIN RASHES

7 JOINT PAIN OR SWELLING

MENSTRUATION

   periods (length, cycle,
     heaviness)
   last period
   menopause
   post-menopausal
     bleeding
   contraception

9  NEUROLOGICAL

   headaches
   fits, faints
   eyes
   ears

anxiety, depression
sleep

10  RISK FACTORS

   medication
   drug abuse
   tobacco
   alcohol
   allergies
   occupational hazards
   foreign travel
   pets

11  OBSTETRIC HISTORY

## FAMILY HISTORY

Record medical problems and causes of death in all first degree
relatives (i.e. parents, siblings and children). If relevant, ask
about problems similar to the patient's which occur in other
relatives.
Record the family history as a family tree, thus:

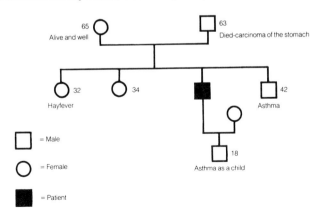

## SOCIAL HISTORY

The social history is very important in understanding not just the disease but the whole patient and how his illness affects him. It may explain why a patient presents at a particular time with a symptom that has been evident for many months.

Some of the questions which you will ask in the social history and the routine review are about very personal matters which the patient would not normally discuss. Answers are more likely to be valuable if you and the patient have built up a confident, trusting relationship earlier in the history.

Find out about:

1 **Housing**: Is it adequate? Are there stairs? Are shops near?
2 **Diet**: Is it adequate? It often helps to get the patient to describe a typical day, including diet.
3 **Contact**: Does the patient live alone? Is there contact with relatives and friends?
4 **Occupation, hobbies**: What occupies the patient at home and at work? Are there any risk factors at either? Are there problems with work and the current illness?
5 **Finance**: Details not usually required. Just 'do you have any financial worries?' How will a period of illness affect this?
6 **Sexual**: Are there problems with current sexual relationships? Any homosexual contact?
7 **Anxieties**: Any marital problems or worries in other relationships? Any other worries?

# EXAMINATION

Look for clues from the first time the patient is seen. After the history conduct a systematic examination, explaining briefly what will be done. A full examination involves all systems but the balance will alter with the case. The order of systems may vary with the individual but make sure that each system is examined fully in a routine manner.

Proceed to a systematic examination covering:

1  GENERAL APPEARANCE
2  CARDIOVASCULAR SYSTEM
3  RESPIRATORY SYSTEM
4  GASTROINTESTINAL SYSTEM
5  NERVOUS SYSTEM
6  BREASTS
7  RETICULO-ENDOTHELIAL SYSTEM
8  THYROID
9  MUSCULOSKELETAL SYSTEM
10  SKIN

# GENERAL APPEARANCE

1 **Signs of distress**: decide how ill the patient is. Does he need urgent treatment before a full examination?
2 **Hydration**: thirst, oliguria, dry skin and tongue, tachycardia, postural hypotension.
3 **Cyanosis**: an increase in deoxygenated haemoglobin—*peripheral*—increased oxygen extraction secondary to poor perfusion or *central*—lung disease or right to left shunt.
4 **Anaemia**: look at conjunctiva inside lower eyelid. Not reliable unless anaemia is gross.
5 **Jaundice**: best seen in sclera while examining the eyes.
6 **Clubbing**: loss of angle between nail and nailbed, then increased nail curvature. Seen in cardiovascular conditions (cyanotic congenital heart disease, infective endocarditis), respiratory disease (bronchogenic carcinoma, fibrosing alveolitis, pus in chest or pleural cavity) and gastrointestinal disease (alcoholic cirrhosis, malabsorption).

# CARDIOVASCULAR SYSTEM

Build up a routine order of examination:

1 GENERAL FEATURES
2 PULSES AND BLOOD PRESSURE
3 JUGULAR VEINS
4 OBSERVATION AND PALPATION OF PRAECORDIUM
5 AUSCULTATION

## GENERAL FEATURES

**Cyanosis, clubbing, anaemia** (p. 10)
**Perfusion**: look for peripheral cyanosis and cool extremities indicating poor cardiac output. Temperature difference between core and periphery.
**Splinter haemorrhages:** thin linear haemorrhages in the long axis of the fingernails, a feature of infective endocarditis.
**Oedema**: fluid in interstitial tissue, usually in ankles or sacrum if patient confined to bed. Push firmly over a bony prominence for ten to fifteen seconds and look for a maintained pit.

## PULSES

**Radial pulse**: feel for rate and rhythm. If irregular, look for a background regular pulse with superimposed ectopic beats or the complete irregularity in time and force of atrial fibrillation. Regular alternating ectopic beats produce pulsus bigeminus. A regular pulse with alternating strong and weak beats, pulsus alternans, may occur in heart failure. Feel radial and femoral pulses together for radiofemoral delay indicating aortic obstruction in coarctation.

**Carotid pulse**: assess the pulse waveform at the carotid. Feel this medial to the midpoint of the sternomastoid. A slow rising pulse is found in aortic stenosis. A fast rising pulse with large pulse pressures and fast fall is found in aortic regurgitation. A decrease in pulse pressure on inspiration occurs in pulsus paradoxus (pericardial effusion or constriction, acute asthma).

**Other pulses**: assess the peripheral vascular system by feeling femoral, popliteal, posterior tibial and dorsalis pedis arteries (*A Surgical Catechism*, pp. 32, 33).

## BLOOD PRESSURE

Measurement of the blood pressure must be part of any routine examination. Make the measurement with the patient relaxed and the arm horizontal, approximately at the level of the heart. Blood pressure in the right arm is around 5 mmHg greater than in the left arm.

Use a sphygmomanometer cuff covering half the upper arm, with all clothing removed from the arm. Inflate the cuff while feeling the radial pulse. The systolic pressure is that pressure at which the pulse disappears. Extend the elbow, find the brachial pulse, place the stethoscope bell gently over the artery and inflate the sphygmomanometer to just above the systolic pressure. Let the column of mercury fall slowly until sounds are just heard (systolic pressure). As it continues to fall the sounds will muffle (Korotkoff phase IV) then disappear (phase V). Phase V is usually taken as diastolic pressure.

### Pulsus paradoxus
In constrictive pericarditis, acute asthma and cardiac tamponade from pericardial effusion, the systolic blood pressure drops on inspiration. A drop of around 5 mmHg is normal on deep inspiration.

Allow the mercury column to drop very slowly as the patient breathes in and out. Sounds will appear first only on expiration, then throughout respiration. The difference between the two levels is the degree of paradoxus.

### Postural hypotension
If fluid depletion is suspected, the patient has postural symptoms or takes antihypertensive drugs, the blood pressures lying and standing are recorded.

## JUGULAR VENOUS PULSE

The jugular veins form a manometer reflecting right atrial filling. Set the backrest at 45 degrees. The internal jugular veins run up between the two heads of the sternomastoid and the external jugular veins run over the muscle. Measure the *vertical* height of the pulsating column above the manubriosternal angle (angle of Louis).

If the veins are not visible, check that they fill with abdominal pressure or the Valsalva manoeuvre.

If veins are full and not pulsatile look for local obstruction, very high atrial pressure or superior vena caval obstruction.

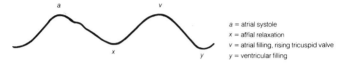

a = atrial systole
x = atrial relaxation
v = atrial filling, rising tricuspid valve
y = ventricular filling

Normal venous waveform

### Abnormalities in jugular veins

1 Obstruction: local or superior vena cava
2 Raised: high atrial pressure
3 Absent *a* wave: atrial fibrillation
4 Large *v* waves: tricuspid regurgitation
5 Intermittent large waves: cannon waves of complete heart block.

## PRAECORDIUM

With the backrest at 45 degrees, look at the front of the chest for scars, symmetry and visible pulsation.
Feel for:

1 **Apex beat**: the guide to the left heart border. The outermost, lowermost point any pulsation is palpable. Start palpating in midaxillary line; define position by ribspace and reference to clavicle or axilla. May be impalpable in obesity or chronic lung disease.
2 **Heaves**: a prominent impulse just medial to the apex (left

ventricular heave) or at the sternal edge (right ventricular heave).
3 **Thrills**: palpable murmurs, usually systolic. Note timing and position.
4 **Sounds**: the 'tapping' apex beat in mitral stenosis is a loud first sound. Extra sounds (e.g. fourth) may be palpable.

## AUSCULTATION

Before starting to listen, review any abnormal findings in the examination so far. See if they point to any particular lesion to which you will need to pay special attention.

Start listening at the apex beat with the bell of the stethoscope resting gently on the chest wall. Listen all over the praecordium, using the diaphragm over the sternum and aortic area.

The stethoscope bell is best for low pitched sounds such as mitral stenosis murmurs, and the diaphragm for high frequency sounds like aortic regurgitation. Use a good stethoscope with snugly fitting ear pieces.

Identify the heart sounds and time all murmurs by feeling the carotid pulse during auscultation. The carotid upstroke comes fractionally after the first heart sound.

*Heart sounds*

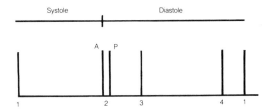

**First sound**: mitral and tricuspid closure. Loud in mitral stenosis, high output, tachycardia. Soft in bradycardia, first degree heart block. Variable in atrial fibrillation, complete heart block.

**Second sound**: aortic and pulmonary closure in that order. Split widens on inspiration. Wide fixed split in atrial septal defect. Paradoxical splitting, pulmonary then aortic in left bundle branch block, hypertension, left heart failure.

**Third sound**: occurs early in diastole, low pitched. Common and normal in children, but in adults signifies rapid ventricular filling, as in mitral regurgitation, or an increase in myocardial tone in the failing ventricle.

**Fourth sound**: occurs late in diastole, caused by atrial contraction. Usually signifies pressure overload, as in hypertension or aortic stenosis. Also hypertrophic obstructive cardiomyopathy.

### Murmurs

Listen all over the praecordium. Check the timing of any murmur with reference to the carotid pulse. If *systolic*, decide whether it runs right through to drown the second sound (pansystolic) or whether it is midsystolic only (ejection).

Pansystolic murmurs occur between high and low pressure systems (mitral regurgitation, VSD). Ejection systolic murmurs occur with two high pressure systems (aortic stenosis).

*Diastolic* murmurs start immediately from the second sound (aortic regurgitation) or are delayed until the atrioventricular valves open (mitral stenosis). Listen for an opening snap as the mitral valve opens. This implies a high left atrial pressure but disappears if the valve calcifies.

Assess the radiation of any murmur (aortic to carotids, mitral to axilla), and the effect of respiration. Left heart murmurs are louder on expiration, right on inspiration.

Mitral murmurs are louder with the patient rolled to the left, and after exercise. Aortic murmurs are louder with the patient sitting up and leaning forward.

Areas of maximum intensity are:

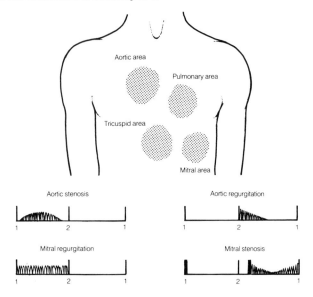

## SYMPTOMS AND SIGNS OF COMMON CONDITIONS

LEFT HEART FAILURE
tiredness, breathlessness
orthopnoea, p.n.d.
poor perfusion
pulsus alternans
added heart sounds
late inspiratory crackles

INFECTIVE ENDOCARDITIS
changing murmurs
splinter haemorrhages
finger clubbing
Osler's nodes
large spleen
Roth's spots in fundi
microscopic haematuria

MITRAL REGURGITATION
tiredness
shortness of breath
atrial fibrillation
displaced apex
pansystolic murmur
third heart sound
ECG changes
large heart on chest X-ray

RIGHT HEART FAILURE
ankle oedema
raised jvp
large tender liver

MITRAL STENOSIS
tiredness
pulmonary oedema
malar flush
atrial fibrillation
palpable first sound
opening snap
mid diastolic murmur
presystolic accentuation
   (not in AF)
loud pulmonary second sound
right ventricular heave
ECG changes
big left atrium on chest X-ray

TRICUSPID REGURGITATION
right heart failure
large *v* wave in jvp
large pulsatile liver
right ventricular heave
pansystolic murmur

AORTIC STENOSIS
chest pain
shortness of breath
faintness on exercise
slow rising pulse
left ventricular heave
ejection systolic murmur
soft aortic second sound
fourth heart sound
LVH on ECG

AORTIC REGURGITATION
shortness of breath
fast rising pulse
displaced apex beat
early diastolic murmur
mid diastolic murmur (Austin-Flint)
large heart on chest X-ray

## ELECTROCARDIOGRAPHY

Changes in electrical potential produced during cardiac contraction are recorded at the body surface. A limb lead is attached to each wrist and ankle, and praecordial leads are attached as shown in the diagrams.

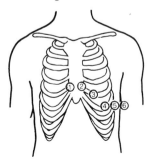

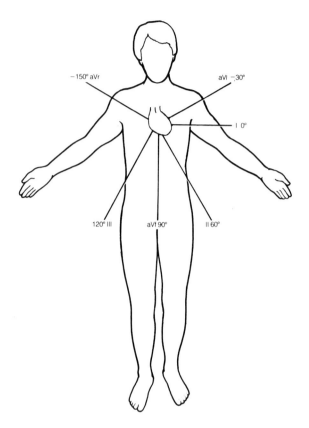

Leads I, II and III are standard bipolar leads connecting inputs from two limbs while aVr, aVl and aVf are unipolar limb leads. These six leads look at the heart from different directions in the frontal plane. They reflect activity in different areas of the heart, and the overall electrical axis can be calculated relevant to this 'hexaxial' system. Lead I is taken as 0 degrees, aVf as + 90 degrees and aVl as −30 degrees.

Standard leads:

 anterolateral heart: aVl, I
 inferior surface: II, III, aVf
 ventricular cavities: aVr

The praecordial leads look around the myocardium. In cross section they appear:

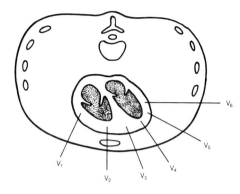

The basic ECG pattern consists of:

P wave: atrial activation
QRS complex: ventricular activation
T wave: ventricular recovery
U wave: further repolarisation
Q wave: negative deflection initiating QRS
S wave: any other negative deflection
PR interval: normal < 0.20 seconds
QRS interval: normal < 0.12 seconds

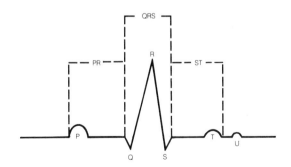

Usual paper speed is 25 mm per second. At this speed one large square on ECG paper (5 mm) is 0.20 seconds.

### Interpretation of the ECG
1 Check name, date, paper speed and calibration
2 Check rate and rhythm
3 Check PR interval, QRS complex
4 Look at P wave size and shape (lead II)
5 Look at QRS throughout
6 Look at ST segment, T waves.

## CONDUCTION

sinus rhythm

atrial fibrillation

atrial flutter (3 : 1)

first degree heart block

second degree heart block

complete heart block

left bundle branch block

right bundle branch block

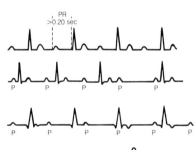

## MYOCARDIAL INFARCTION

Signs:
1 Q waves
2 ST elevation
3 T wave inversion

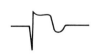

Site:
Inferior       =   II, III, aVf
Anteroseptal   =   I, $V_2$–$V_4$
Anterolateral  =   I, aVl, $V_5$, $V_6$
Posterior      =   inverted signs in $V_1$

## RADIOLOGY OF THE HEART

On standard postero-anterior chest X-rays, the transverse
diameter of the heart should be less than half the transverse
thoracic diameter. The only chamber enlargement which can be
diagnosed with any confidence is left atrial enlargement when
the atrial appendage bulges out below the main pulmonary
artery and a double shadow appears at the right heart border.

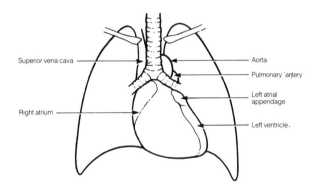

# RESPIRATORY SYSTEM

## GENERAL EXAMINATION

Examine the respiratory system with the patient lying comfortably in bed, chest exposed, and backrest at 45 degrees. Look for:

1 **Respiratory distress**: fast breathing rate, gasping respiration, audible wheeze
2 **Cyanosis** (p. 10)
3 **Clubbing** (p. 10)
4 **Flapping tremor**: a coarse tremor of the hands, accentuated by wrist extension. Usually signifies $CO_2$ retention
5 **Chest shape**: asymmetry, scars, big antero-posterior diameter (barrel chest).

Carry out the full examination on the front of the chest, then help the patient to sit up and repeat it on the back.

Get used to a routine of:  observation
palpation
percussion
auscultation.

Compare the two sides and move gradually down the chest. Never forget to examine the lateral aspects with the front of the chest.

## OBSERVATION

Observe the respiratory rate and rhythm without drawing the patient's attention to his breathing. The normal rate is 15 to 20 per minute.
Look for:

1 **Fast rate**: fast and shallow in restrictive disease, prolonged expiration with obstruction.

2 **Periodic respiration** (Cheyne-Stokes breathing): regular waxing and waning of depth, often with apnoea.
3 **Use of accessory muscles**: sternomastoids, scalenes.
4 **Abdominal movement**: inward movement on inspiration suggests diaphragm weakness.
5 **Symmetry**: stand at the foot of the bed and compare the movement of the two sides of the chest.

## PALPATION

### Mediastinum
**Trachea**: assess the position of the upper mediastinum by feeling the trachea in the suprasternal notch. Feel for deviation from the midline as the trachea enters the thorax. Do this with the patient sitting up, neck muscles relaxed.
**Apex beat**: movement of the apex beat may be a sign of cardiac pathology or changes in the surrounding lung.

### Expansion
Measure expansion in upper, then lower zones. Spread the fingers wide and ask the patient to take a maximum inspiration.

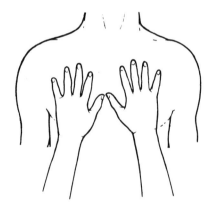

### Tactile Vocal Fremitus (TVF)
Feel for transmitted vibration with the flat of the hand while the patient repeats '99'. TVF is decreased by collapse, pleural fluid and pneumothorax, but increased by the improved conduction through consolidated lung, i.e. pneumonia.

## PERCUSSION

The middle digit of one hand percusses on the middle phalanx of the middle digit of the other hand applied firmly to the chest. Use one or two percussion strokes at each point. At the apices percussion may be directly on the clavicles.

Listen for the percussion note and feel the vibration in the percussed finger.

Compare the two sides:

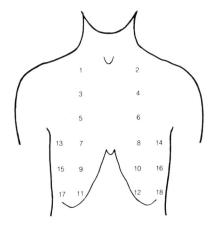

The percussion note is dull when the underlying lung is consolidated, collapsed or fibrosed, and very dull over pleural fluid.

## AUSCULTATION

Using bell or diaphragm, listen in all the areas you percussed. Ask the patient to open his mouth and breathe. This usually provokes a suitable increase in tidal volume.

In normal breath sounds, inspiration is heard with very little in expiration. Bronchial breathing consists of blowing sounds heard through inspiration and expiration with a slight silent pause between the two. Bronchial breathing is heard over consolidated lung and over trachea and right main bronchus. Voice sounds are also better transmitted over consolidated lung and even whispers are well heard (whispering pectoriloquy).

Added sounds are of three sorts:

1 **Wheezes**: continuous musical sounds caused by narrowed airways, mostly expiratory, usually multiple. A single fixed wheeze suggests large airway obstruction.
2 **Crackles**: interrupted sounds caused by airway opening. Early inspiratory in chronic bronchitis and emphysema. Late inspiratory in fibrosing alveolitis and pulmonary oedema. Coarse and at any time in bronchiectasis.
3 **Pleural rubs**: often creaking or grating, inspiration or expiration.

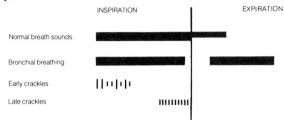

## PATTERNS OF ABNORMALITY

It is often difficult to be confident of a respiratory sign in isolation. Build up a pattern as you examine the chest.

|  | Pneumo-thorax | Collapse | Fibrosis | Consoli-dation | Pleural Fluid | Airflow Obstruction |
|---|---|---|---|---|---|---|
| Mediastinum | moves away in tension pneumothorax | towards lesion | towards lesion | central | may move away | central |
| Expansion | reduced | reduced | reduced | reduced | reduced | reduced overinflation |
| Vocal fremitus | reduced | reduced | increased | increased | reduced | reduced |
| Percussion | increased resonance | dull | dull | dull | stony dull | reduced, cardiac dullness |
| Auscultation | reduced breath sounds | reduced breath sounds | crackles, may be bronchial breathing | bronchial breathing | reduced sounds | early crackles, prolonged expiration |

## SPUTUM

It is not normal to cough up sputum. Always examine sputum carefully. Look for:

1 **Colour**: yellow or green usually means infection, occasionally eosinophilia. Blood in the sputum (haemoptysis) usually requires further investigation.
2 **Plugs**: hard plugs may be produced in asthma. Teased out, they may show casts of the airways. Firm brownish plugs occur in allergic bronchopulmonary aspergillosis.

## BEDSIDE RESPIRATORY FUNCTION TESTS

Simple bedside respiratory function tests are part of the assessment of any breathless patient. Learn to use a peak flow meter and a spirometer. Normal values vary with age, height, sex and race.

*Peak Expiratory Flow Rate*: Measures maximum flow in a short, sharp expiration. Use a Wright's peak flow meter or mini peak flow meter.

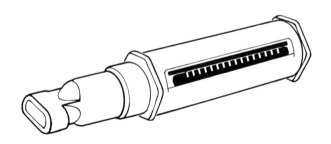

*Spirometry*: Usually done on a Vitallograph dry bellows spirometer during a forced maximal expiration. The ratio $FEV_1/FVC$ (forced expiratory ratio) should be around 75%. It is low in airflow obstruction but not in restrictive diseases (e.g. fibrosing alveolitis) despite reduced FVC.

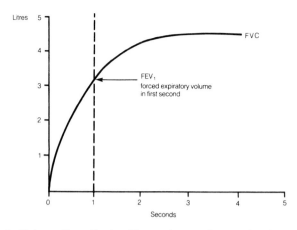

*Minute Volume*: In patients with respiratory depression (e.g. drug overdose) monitor the volume breathed in one minute with a Wright's respirometer attached to a face mask.

## CHEST X-RAY

Learn the normal landmarks on postero-anterior and lateral films. Look at the X-ray in a routine order:

1 Name, date, information on type of X-ray (supine, etc.)
2 Centering (look at clavicular heads and vertebral spines)
3 The heart shadow (p. 21)
4 The lung fields for size, diffuse opacities, nodular shadows, cavities, fissures
5 The mediastinum and hila, especially aorta and trachea
6 The bones, particularly ribs but also vertebrae, humeri, scapulae
7 Soft tissues.

Describe the position and characteristics of all abnormalities using simple terms. Avoid terms with distinct pathological associations. For this purpose divide the lung fields into upper, middle and lower zones, defined by anterior ends of second and fourth ribs. Precise anatomical location usually requires a lateral.

# THE GASTROINTESTINAL SYSTEM

First look for jaundice (p. 10) and the signs of chronic liver disease. Examine the oropharynx, then lie the patient down comfortably with one pillow to examine the abdomen. Signs of chronic liver disease are:

1 Palmar erythema
2 White nails
3 Clubbing
4 Spider naevi
5 Gynaecomastia
6 Testicular atrophy.

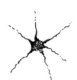

Spider naevus –
dilated central arteriole
controls filling

Look at the oropharynx for:

1 Angular cheilitis, soreness at the corners of the mouth
2 Hydration (tongue dry or moist)
3 Smooth tongue (iron, $B_{12}$ deficiency)
4 Ulcers
5 Buccal pigmentation (Addison's disease, racial)
6 Condition of teeth and gums.

Abdominal examination:

1 Make sure the patient is warm, comfortable and relaxed.
2 Note any scars or obvious masses.
3 Gently palpate the four quadrants of the abdomen looking for tenderness and masses.
4 Palpate deeper in each quadrant.
5 If you detect any masses record the size, surface, consistency, movement with respiration, pulsation, tenderness.
6 Feel specifically for liver, spleen and kidneys.

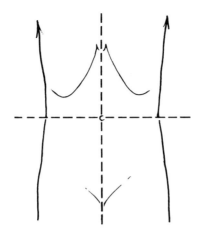

## LIVER

The liver is detected by feeling the descent of the lower edge
with respiration using the tips of the index and middle fingers.
Start at the umbilicus and keep firm downward pressure during a
deep respiration. Move quickly up under the right costal margin.

Percuss the vertical height of the liver dullness in the
midclavicular line (should be less than 13 cm).

If the liver is palpable, assess:

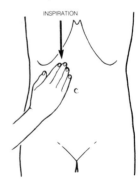

Vertical height of dullness
Extent below costal margin
Consistency (soft, firm or hard)
Edge (smooth, irregular)
Surface (smooth, nodular)
Tenderness
Pulsation
Presence of bruit (auscultate)

## SPLEEN

Examine for the movement of the spleen with respiration in the
same way as the liver. Start around the umbilicus and move up
under the left costal margin.

The spleen is distinguished from a large left kidney by the fact that the kidney is bimanually palpable and the spleen is dull to percussion anteriorly.

It is often easier to feel a mildly enlarged spleen by turning the patient on to the right side.

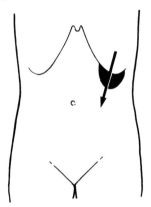

## KIDNEYS

Try to feel the kidneys by deep palpation between two hands placed anteriorly and posteriorly. The lower pole of the right kidney may be palpable in thin normal subjects. Normal left kidneys are not palpable.

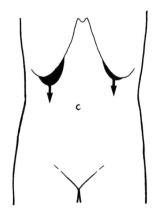

## GROINS

Examine the groins for lymph nodes and for hernias (*A Surgical Catechism*, pp. 14, 15).

## ASCITES

Look for evidence of peritoneal fluid by examining for shifting dullness. Percuss into the flanks with the patient supine. If the flanks are dull to percussion, mark the upper limit of dullness, then ask the patient to turn onto the opposite side and percuss again. Ascites moves around in the abdomen with gravity and the level of dullness to percussion shifts accordingly.

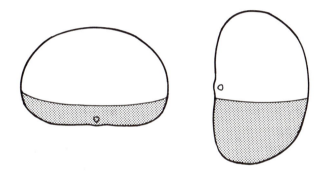

## GENITALIA

It is all too easy to omit examination of the genitalia to save your own or the patient's embarrassment.

Look at the penis for evidence of ulceration. Examine the scrotal contents. Common swellings are:

1 **Hernia** in scrotal sac
2 **Hydrocoele**: difficult to feel testis, swelling transilluminates
3 **Epididymo-orchitis**: inflamed, tender, swollen
4 **Varicocoele**: 'bag of worms' around testis
5 **Spermatocoele**: separable from testis
6 **Testicular tumour.**
7 **Epididymal cyst**.

*Rectal Examination*

Explain what is to be done and why. Ask the patient to turn on to the left side with knees curled up. Examine the perianal skin. Lubricate your gloved index finger and exert steady pressure on the anal orifice to insert the finger into the rectum.

Feel all around the rectum. In the male, delineate the size, surface and consistency of the prostate gland. If any masses are felt, they can often be distinguished further by palpating between the finger in the rectum and a hand on the anterior abdominal wall.

## NUTRITION AND HYDRATION

Signs of marked weight loss may be obvious as redundant folds of skin. Other degrees of nutritional problems may show as specific signs, e.g. spoon-shaped nails (koilonychia) in iron deficiency or smooth tongue in iron or $B_{12}$ deficiency.

Hydration is often difficult to assess. Look for:

1 **Sunken eyes**
2 **Poor tissue turgor**: pick up a fold of skin and see how quickly it springs back (unreliable in old people)
3 **Dry tongue** (may occur with mouth breathing)
4 **Postural hypotension**.

# THE NERVOUS SYSTEM

A full neurological examination requires a great deal of time and effort on the part of the patient and examiner. It also requires some knowledge of neuroanatomy in order to interpret the findings. In some situations it is acceptable to perform an abbreviated neurological examination which can be extended if abnormalities are found.

Throughout the examination try to pick out the pattern of any abnormal findings and how they relate to each other. You will need to examine:

1 **Higher functions and speech**
2 **Cranial nerves**
3 **Motor system**—observation
               —tone
               —power
               —reflexes
               —co-ordination
4 **Sensory system**—touch
               —pain, temperature
               —vibration, joint position sense
5 **Gait**

## HIGHER FUNCTIONS, SPEECH

Much of the necessary information will have been gathered during the history taking.

### Level of consciousness

Depression of consciousness is graded:

1 Drowsy, rousable and responding appropriately
2 Some spontaneous movements, responds to pain, strong lights, loud noise
3 Responds to pain by withdrawal
4 No spontaneous movement, no response to any stimuli

If conscious level is normal, test orientation in time and space.

### Memory
**Long term memory** will be evident from the history.
**Short term memory**: 'digit span'—the patient should be able to repeat six or seven numbers. Test with a name and address repeated five minutes later.

### Speech
**Dysarthria**: a problem with the motor production of voice sounds.
**Dysphasia**: impaired understanding or expression of language:
> —expressive:explaining (temporo-parietal)
> —receptive:understanding (posterior parietal)
> —nominal:naming objects (temporal)

## CRANIAL NERVES

### 1 Olfactory
Loss of smell is usually related to nasal problems. Ensure patency, then test each nostril separately with a common, mild odour (orange, coffee).

### 2 Optic
Visual acuity—use a Snellen chart at 6 metres. Test near vision with Jaeger cards and colour vision with Ishihara cards.

**Visual fields**: these are assessed roughly by confrontation. Sit opposite the patient on the same level. Assess the outer range of each eye separately by moving a white pinhead in a plane half way between you and the patient. Compare your field with the patient's.

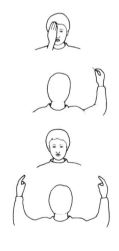

With both eyes open, test the patient's ability to detect finger movements in upper and lower outer quadrants, moving one finger, then both together. The most common defect in hospital patients is a homonymous hemianopia after a cerebrovascular accident. A minor defect may show only as inattention on one side when both fingers move.

**Ophthalmoscope**: learn to use an ophthalmoscope to examine fundus, lens, cornea and the chambers of the eye.

### 3, 4 and 6 Oculomotor, trochlear, abducens
The oculomotor supplies all eye muscles except superior oblique (4) and lateral rectus (6). It also supplies levator palpebrae superioris and parasympathetic fibres for accommodation and pupil constriction.

1 Look for ptosis (drooping of upper eyelid) and test pupil response to light (move light onto pupil from outside direction of gaze) and accommodation.
2 Ask the patient to follow steady finger movement to right and left, up and down with head still. Ask about diplopia (double vision) during this test. Look for nystagmus (rhythmic oscillations of the eyes, usually with slow drift and fast return). Nystagmus is caused by vestibular abnormalities, cerebellar lesions, drugs (phenytoin) or very poor visual acuity.
3 Look for squint: *non paralytic*—difference in optical axis maintained throughout movements, often no diplopia. *Paralytic*—related to muscle weakness, occurs (with diplopia) in direction of muscle action.
4 Examine for Horner's Syndrome: a cervical sympathetic lesion causing:
—ptosis
—small pupil
—eye indrawn (enophthalmos)
—lack of sweating over half of face

### 5 Trigeminal
Sensory supply to face including cornea and motor supply to muscles of mastication. Feel temporal and masseter muscles with teeth clenched. Test sensation to touch and pinprick in each division.

Test the corneal reflex with a piece of cotton wool with a distinct end that you can control. With the patient looking away from you, touch the cornea (not sclera). Look for a blink reflex and ask the patient to compare sensation on the two sides.

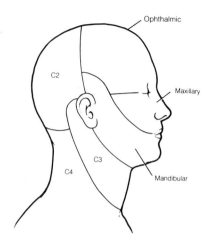

Ophthalmic

Maxillary

Mandibular

C2

C3

C4

### 7 Facial

Supplies all face and scalp muscles except mastication (5) and levator palpebrae superioris (3). Also travels with chorda tympani carrying taste from anterior two thirds of the tongue. Look for facial symmetry as patient smiles, shows his teeth, shuts his eyes and raises his eyebrows.

Upper motor neurone facial lesions (supranuclear) spare the forehead (bilaterally represented). Lower motor neurone lesions involve the whole face. Facial canal lesions produce loss of taste and paralysis of stapedius which gives hyperacusis on the affected side.

### 8 Vestibulocochlear

**Vestibular**: the patient may complain of vertigo. Look for nystagmus (p. 35).

**Cochlear**: test hearing by covering one ear and whispering number 3 m from other ear. Compare air and bone conduction by Rinne's test. Hold a lightly vibrating tuning fork (256 cycles/s) at the external auditory meatus, then on the mastoid bone. If it is louder on the bone, bone conduction is better than air conduction; middle ear disease is the usual cause.

In Weber's test, the tuning fork is placed in the centre of the forehead. Nerve conduction defects on one side produce lateralisation to the other ear.

### 9 Glossopharyngeal

Sensory supply to posterior pharynx, posterior third of tongue and part of the external ear canal. Test the gag reflex by touching posterior pharyngeal wall on each side with an orange stick. Look for pharyngeal constriction and palatal elevation. If there is no movement ask about sensation (sensory limb is glossopharyngeal, motor is vagus). For taste, ask the patient to put out his tongue. Rub the appropriate dried area with sugar, salt or an effervescent vitamin C tablet. The patient raises his hand on tasting it. Test each side, front and back before the patient puts his tongue back in.

### 10 Vagus

Look for the motor element of the gag reflex and listen for dysarthria (including the weak voice with inability to cough found with a recurrent laryngeal nerve lesion).

### 11 Spinal accessory

Supplies sternomastoid and trapezius muscles. Test sternomastoids together by pushing the head forward against resistance, or individually by resisted chin rotation. Test trapezius by asking the patient to shrug his shoulders against resistance.

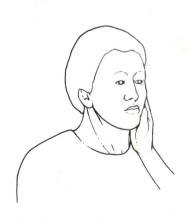

Contraction of right sternomastoid with resisted rotation to the left.

### 12 Hypoglossal

Look at the tongue lying in the floor of the mouth. A lower motor neurone lesion will produce wasting and fasciculation (fine spontaneous muscle fibre contraction) on one side, while an upper motor neurone lesion produces a stiff bulky tongue. Ask the patient to put the tongue in and out. It will deviate towards the side of any muscle weakness.

## MOTOR SYSTEM

### Observation

Expose the limbs and look for:

**Position**: e.g. flexed arm of hemiplegia.

**Muscle wasting**: examine particularly small hand muscles.

**Fasciculation**: fine spontaneous fibre contractions found in lower motor neurone lesions.

**Involuntary movements**: gross movements or tremor which may be:

—fine (thyrotoxicosis, anxiety)

—slow, coarse (Parkinson's disease)

—flapping ($CO_2$ retention)

—on movement (intention tremor of cerebellar disease).

### Tone

The sensation of resistance felt on passive movement of a joint in a relaxed patient.

Take the patient's hand as if to shake it and passively move the elbow looking for rigidity. Make a quick supination movement to look for spasticity, which is felt as a catch and then release, like a clasp knife.

In the leg, roll the extended leg for rigidity. For spasticity, suddenly flex the knee. A spastic catch will kick the foot off the bed.

**Hypotonia** is difficult to detect.

**Rigidity** occurs with extrapyramidal lesions. Tone is increased throughout all movement at a joint. It feels like bending a stiff lead pipe and may have a superimposed tremor (cogwheel).

**Spasticity** is a sign of upper motor neurone lesions.

## Power

In routine testing, select a number of movements to test.
Isometric testing, trying to push the patient out of a demonstrated position, is rather easier for patients to understand.
Grade power:

0 = no active contraction
1 = visible, palpable contraction; no movement
2 = movement with gravity eliminated
3 = movement against gravity
4 = movement against gravity and resistance but weak
5 = normal power.

Compare power on the two sides. The scheme shown should bring out most abnormalities and is quickly performed.

| Movement | Muscle | Nerve | Nerve Root |
|---|---|---|---|
| UPPER LIMB | | | |
| 1 shoulder abduction | deltoid | circumflex | C5 |
| 2 elbow flexion (forearm supinated) | biceps | musculo-cutaneous | (C5) C6 |
| 3 elbow extension | triceps | radial | C7 |
| 4 finger extension | extensor digitorum | radial | C7, C8 |
| 5 finger flexion | flexor digitorum sublimus | median | C8 |
| | flexor digitorum profundus | median + ulnar | |
| 6 thumb abduction | abductor pollicis brevis | median | T1 |
| 7 little finger abduction | first dorsal interosseus | ulnar | T1 |
| LOWER LIMB | | | |
| 1 hip flexion | ilio-psoas | femoral | L2, 3 |
| 2 knee extension | quadriceps | femoral | L3, L4 |
| 3 hip extension | gluteus maximus | inferior gluteal | L5, S1 |
| 4 knee flexion | hamstrings | sciatic | L5, S1 |
| 5 ankle dorsiflexion | tibialis anterior | sciatic | L4 |
| 6 great toe dorsiflexion | extensor hallucis longus | sciatic | L5 |
| 7 ankle plantar flexion | gastrocnemius | sciatic | S1, S2 |

If any weakness is detected, try to work out the pattern. Is it pyramidal, nerve root, peripheral nerve, etc? (More detailed information on peripheral nerve examination can be found in '*Aids to Investigation of Peripheral Nerve Injuries*', HMSO, London).

### Reflexes
Reflexes are reduced by lower motor neurone lesions and increased by upper motor neurone lesions, sometimes with clonus. Compare reflexes on the two sides. Use a long handled reflex hammer and develop a consistent technique. Place both limbs symmetrically and apply the same stimulus to both sides.

| Reflex | Nerve Root | Position |
|---|---|---|
| Biceps | C5, C6 | elbow flexed 60 degrees |
| Supinator | C6 | elbow flexed, between supination and pronation |
| Triceps | C7 | elbow flexed 90 degrees |
| Finger | C8 | fingers extended at mcp, flexed at xip joints |
| Knee | L3, L4 | knee flexed 30 degrees and supported |
| Ankle | L5, S1 | hip externally rotated, knee flexed 30 degrees, ankle 90 degrees. |

If reflexes are absent try to bring them out with reinforcement, repeating the reflex while the patient contracts another muscle hard, e.g. clenching the fists.

**Clonus**: sudden sustained stretching of a muscle may produce oscillating contraction and relaxation, a sign of an upper motor neurone lesion.

### Superficial reflexes
**Abdominal reflexes**: stimulated by stroking the skin with an orange stick. This produces contraction of anterior abdominal wall muscles. Absent in upper motor neurone lesions but also with a fat abdomen.

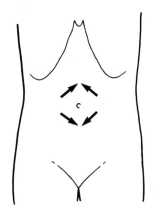

**Plantar reflex**: scratch an orange stick or key firmly along the outer edge of the sole of the foot. Look for the first movement of the great toe. Upper motor neurone lesions produce extension with fanning and extension of other toes.

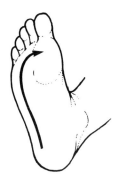

*Co-ordination*

Co-ordination requires integration of power and tone of muscles, muscle spindles, joint receptors and cerebellar function. Tests of co-ordination are mostly used to assess cerebellar function.

**Finger nose test**: ask the patient to move his index finger quickly and accurately between his nose and your finger. The two fingers should make contact near the limit of the patient's reach. In cerebellar ataxia the movements become clumsy at the limits—intention tremor.

**Heel shin test**: ask the patient to raise one leg straight off the bed to 30 degrees, then place the heel on the opposite knee and run it quickly and accurately down the shin.

**Dysdiadochokinesia**: rapidly alternating movements such as tapping with hand or foot are disturbed in cerebellar disease.

## SENSORY SYSTEM

Compare similar areas on two sides of the body. It is usually enough to test just three sensations: touch, pinprick and vibration or joint position.

Learn the distribution of appropriate dermatomes and peripheral nerves. Test sensation in each limb, moving down through the dermatomes.

ANTERIOR

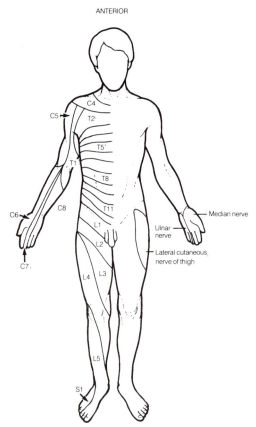

POSTERIOR

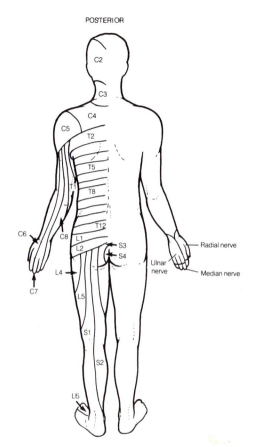

**Touch**: cotton wool or gentle finger pressure. Give one distinct stimulus, not a stroke.

**Pain**: use a pin for superficial pain. Make sure the patient recognises the sharp sensation, not just pressure. Deep pain can be tested by squeezing the Achilles' tendon.

**Temperature**: test quickly with a cold object (e.g. tuning fork). Formal testing involves tubes of hot and cold water.

**Vibration**: press a vibrating 128 Hz tuning fork over bony prominences, starting at the malleoli. The patient must detect vibration, not just pressure.

43

**Joint position**: hold the terminal phalanx with finger and thumb on medial and lateral sides. Make small but distinct movements up or down. In the fingers, the patient should be able to sense very small movements. If vibration and joint position sense are intact peripherally, there is no need to test proximally.

### Scheme for sensory testing

Start on the face, move to the shoulders and down the arms by dermatomes. Use light touch and pinprick and compare the two arms. Then look at joint position sense in the fingers. Repeat the procedure in the legs.

### Meningeal irritation

This is most often caused by meningeal infection or by leak of blood into the subarachnoid space.
Test for:

**Neck stiffness**: with one hand on each side of the head flex the neck passively. In meningeal irritation neck muscles will contract to prevent any painful movement.

**Kernig's sign**: most useful in children. With the knee flexed 90 degrees flex the hip, then try to straighten the knee. With meningeal irritation this is resisted because of the back pain.

## GAIT

**Hemiplegia**: extended knee, foot swings in an arc
**Sensory ataxia**: high stepping, stamping gait
**Cerebellar**: wide stance, unsteady, unable to follow a line
**Parkinson's**: bent forwards, slow to start and stop, short, shuffling steps
**Proximal weakness**: waddling, swaying gait.

# BREASTS

With the patient sitting, disrobed to the waist, hands on hips, look carefully for breast asymmetry. Examine the skin for redness, ulceration and localised oedema (peau d'orange). Examine the nipples for retraction and discharge.

Feel the four quadrants of each breast with the flat of the fingers. It may help to repeat this with the patient's hands on her head.

If a lump is palpable, assess:

1 Size
2 Consistency, surface
3 Tenderness
4 Fixation to skin or underlying tissue
5 Draining lymph nodes.

Take the opportunity to teach self examination to the patient.

Males may develop significant, palpable breast tissue (gynaecomastia). It is felt as a distinct disc of tissue rather than the general enlargement of obesity. It is often tender.

Causes of gynaecomastia are:

1 Puberty
2 Drugs (oestrogens, spironolactone)
3 Cirrhosis
4 Bronchial neoplasms
5 Klinefelter's syndrome
6 Choriocarcinoma of testis
7 Carcinoma of breast.

# THE RETICULO-ENDOTHELIAL SYSTEM

In a routine examination look at tonsils and spleen, feel for submandibular, cervical, supraclavicular, axillary, para-aortic and inguinal lymph nodes. Pay particular attention to cervical and supraclavicular areas. Examine from behind with the finger tips. Carefully examine nodes draining any skin or other local lesion.

If nodes are palpable record size, number, consistency and mobility; a sketch often helps.

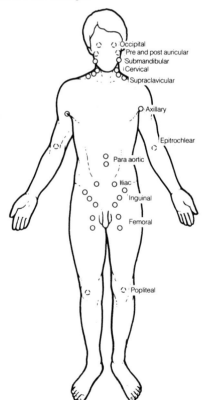

Principal lymph node groups.

# THE THYROID

Look at the neck from the front and then palpate from behind the seated patient. In normal subjects the thyroid is often not palpable. (Test for mobility during swallowing.)

1 Assess thyroid size, symmetry and nodularity.
2 Listen for a bruit.
3 Examine regional lymph nodes.
4 Look for signs of:

**Hypothyroidism**
puffy face
dry skin
coarse hair
hoarse voice
slow pulse
slow relaxing reflexes

**Hyperthyroidism**
fine tremor
sweaty palms
exophthalmos
lid lag
fast pulse
atrial fibrillation
proximal myopathy
pretibial myxoedema

# THE MUSCULOSKELETAL SYSTEM

Assessment of joints consists of observation, palpation and range of movement.

## OBSERVATION

Joint deformity, enlargement, subluxation (partial loss of contact of joint surfaces) and dislocation (complete loss of contact).

In rheumatoid arthritis, common abnormalities are ulnar deviation at metacarpophalangeal joints, swan neck and boutonnière deformities.

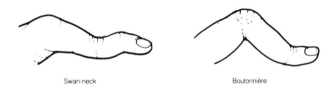

Swan-neck                          Boutonnière

Look for gouty tophi, orangey-yellow in colour around joints and helix of the ear.

Rheumatoid nodules are firm subcutaneous lumps most common at the elbow. Heberden's nodes are bony enlargements at the distal interphalangeal joints in osteoarthritis.

Look for muscle wasting around affected joints. Record the pattern of joint involvement, symmetrical or asymmetrical, small or large joint, weight bearing, etc.

Always look for arteritis, particularly around the nail folds.

## PALPATION

Inflamed joints may be very tender. Differentiate between hard bony swellings, firm synovial tissue thickening and fluctuant fluid. Define areas of tenderness and warmth.

## MOVEMENT

Assess active and passive movement. Measure the movement possible from the neutral position for each joint. This can be done accurately with a goniometer, a sort of modified protractor.

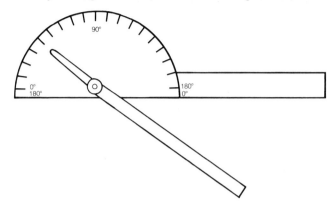

Some conditions produce increased joint mobility (familial, Marfan's syndrome, Ehlers-Danlos syndrome).

When movement is restricted the abnormality may lie in bone, cartilage, synovium, capsule, ligaments, muscles or nerves. Consider each element in turn to find the cause.

### Spine

Kyphosis:concave forwards
Lordosis:convex forwards
Scoliosis:spinal rotation
Cervical spine—examine:
rotation, flexion, extension to
each side, lateral bending
Dorsal and lumbar spine—
examine: flexion, extension,
lateral bending

Sacro-iliac joints—look for:
tenderness on direct pressure
over joint and firm pressure on
anterior iliac crests.

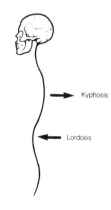

### Shoulder
Abduction
Extension
Flexion
External rotation
Internal rotation

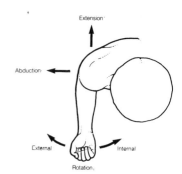

### Elbow
Flexion
Hyperextension
Supination
Pronation

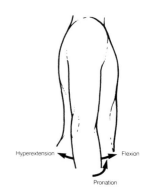

### Wrist
Dorsal flexion
Palmar flexion
Radial deviation
Ulnar deviation

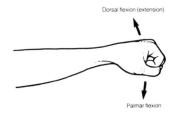

### Fingers
Flexion at metacarpophalangeal and interphalangeal joints

### *Thumb*
Extension
Flexion
Opposition
Abduction

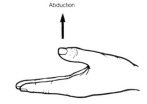

### *Hip*
Flexion
Extension
Rotation in flexion
Rotation in extension

### *Knee*
Flexion
Hyperextension

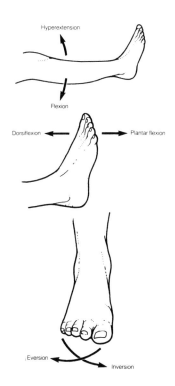

### *Ankle*
Dorsiflexion
Plantar flexion

### *Foot*
Inversion
Eversion

### *Toes*
Flexion and extension at metatarsophalangeal and interphalangeal joints.

# THE SKIN

In the assessment of skin rashes, look at all the skin surface together with the hair, nails and mucous membranes. Note the distribution of any lesions, e.g. light exposed areas.

**Colour**: pigmentation in Addison's disease or patches of depigmentation in vitiligo.
**Eczema**: or dermatitis describes inflammation of the skin.
**Haemorrhage**: skin haemorrhage does not blanch on pressure. *Purpura* describes small areas of haemorrhage, *ecchymosis* widespread haemorrhage or bruising.
**Macules**: impalpable areas of discolouration.
**Papules**: elevations of skin up to 5 mm diameter.
**Nodules**: palpable lesions, larger than papules.
**Vesicles**: fluid-containing lesions up to 5 mm diameter.
**Bullae**: large fluid-filled lesions, blisters.
**Pustules**: vesicles or bullae containing pus.
**Plaques**: well-defined flat areas of abnormal skin, raised or depressed, e.g. psoriasis.
**Wheals**: raised lesions caused by oedema in the dermis.
**Scaling**: abnormal keratinization.
**Fissures**: cracks in epidermis exposing underlying dermis.
**Ulcers**: an area of loss of full thickness of epidermis. Note the condition of the ulcer floor and edge.
**Scars**: examine scars carefully for adequacy of healing, pigmentation (Addison's) or keloid (hypertrophic scars usually in negroid skin).

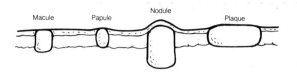

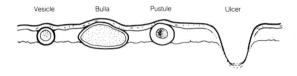

Common skin lesions

# MAKING SENSE OF YOUR FINDINGS

Students often become proficient at taking a history and carrying out an examination but falter when it comes to making sense of the findings and presenting them.

Do not think your job is done when you come to the end of the examination. Go through all the abnormal features you have found and decide whether you need to ask any more questions or perform any further examination.

Then try to put the findings together. Take into account all the features and how they relate to the life of the individual patient. Many doctors find it useful to collate the abnormalities under specific problem headings. For these purposes a problem may be defined as:

1 A proven diagnosis, e.g. carcinoma of the breast
2 A pathological state, e.g. left heart failure
3 An abnormal symptom, sign or investigation, e.g. enlarged spleen
4 A past illness or operation, e.g. rheumatic fever
5 A psychological or social problem, e.g. poor or unsuitable housing
6 A significant risk factor, e.g. smoking.

Whether or not you use fully problem orientated notes will depend largely on the practice in your hospital, but it is always worthwhile gathering your thoughts together in this way initially.

Decide whether a problem needs action in terms of investigations, treatment or explanation, and make plans for such action for each individual problem and their priority. At the end of this process you should have a succinct picture of the patient's problems and a comprehensive plan for the investigations which will be necessary, the treatment which should be started and the information which needs to be given to the patient about his condition.

Patients in hospital need to be seen regularly and

developments recorded in the notes. Note relevant symptoms, signs, investigation results and treatment. Also record any information given to the patient. This is particularly important in the case of patients with malignant disease.

In examination conditions, it is essential to leave five minutes at the end of your long case to sort out the problems and their management. Even if you are running short of time, this is of much greater value than finishing off the last details of the examination.

# PRESENTING YOUR CASE

On ward rounds and examinations, you should present your case concisely, keep to relevant information and bear in mind that the patient may be listening. Start with a sentence introducing the patient and the way he came to medical attention. Then give a detailed history of the present complaint, using the patient's own words whenever possible. Do not put in your own interpretations or diagnoses at this point.

The rest of the history should be an edited version of the information you obtained. Give only relevant details, positive or negative, from the previous medical history, family history, social history and review of systems. If the main complaint is a cough, the absence of shortness of breath should be stated but bowel disturbance can be regarded as absent unless you report any symptoms.

When presenting the examination findings, start with the system primarily affected. Try to be confident in your statements. Do not make excuses for difficulties in the examination without very strong justification. As in the history, present positive findings and important negative findings.

At the end of the examination, pass straight on to a brief summary and your analysis of the problems without further prompting. When giving diagnoses, present the relevant evidence for your interpretation.

Listen to the way in which other doctors present cases on ward rounds and at clinical meetings and pick out the good and bad points. Medical students often feel overwhelmed at first by their lack of knowledge and experience. Read up about the problems you see in your patients, as you are much more likely to remember information if you can relate it to a real person. Using the information you obtain from your patients to sort out problems and commit yourself to diagnoses is the best way to learn.